SCIENTIFIC METHOD IN BIOLOGY.

BY
DR. ELIZABETH BLACKWELL.

INTRODUCTION.

A CONTROVERSY is persistently carried on between an increasing body of the non-professional laity and an important section of the medical profession, in relation to the methods pursued in investigating biological phenomena.

The criticism of medical research by non-medical people is naturally resented by some who are engaged in experimentation; and it is stated seriously that non-scientific persons will impede progress if they interfere with, or succeed in restricting, the efforts of those who specially devote themselves to this branch of research.

This controversy is still going on in ever-widening circles; and it is bound to do so, until the present confusion of thought which exists on this subject is removed, and the broad distinction between right and wrong experimentation is more fully acknowledged and more clearly defined. Our relation to the lower animals has never yet been brought fully into the clear light of reason and conscience. Yet in the order of Providential development it must so come forward.

As advancing humanity has gradually recognised natural rights as existing in the various races of mankind—is carrying on a persistent warfare against human slavery—is slowly awakening to the moral crime of introducing disease and vice amongst native races; and the rights, as well as duties, of women and of children are being gradually recognised; so the time has come when the natural rights of inferior living creatures must be seriously studied.

This study has become obligatory, not only in regard to the welfare of the brute creation, but for the sake of our own human growth as rational and moral beings.

The common-sense of mankind recognises our right to use the lower animals for human benefit, whilst our superior intelligence gives us the power to so use them. But 'can' and 'ought' are different aspects of our mental constitution, which require to he harmonized. What we can do is not the true measure of what we ought to do, in any department of life.

We can starve a child, or lash a horse to death, but we have no right to do so.

The laws of our human constitution compel us to recognise that intellect and conscience, although essential parts, are not identical parts of our nature. Long experience shows us that social progress can only become permanent when conscience guides intelligence.

How far the guidance of conscience can extend, with the practical results to medical research involved in the recognition of such guidance, forms the subject of present consideration.

I.
THE GROWTH OF CONSCIENCE.

IT is through the gradual and harmonious development of intelligence with that element in our nature that we name conscience that the human race passes from lower to higher states of civilization. In pursuing our ideals, conscience is our instinctive monitor of right and wrong.

Our great naturalist, **Darwin**, laid down as a law of evolution that 'the moral sense, or conscience, is by far the most important of the differences between man and the lower animals. Duty—"ought"—is the most noble of all the attributes of man.'

Victor Hugo, with the prophetic insight of genius, calls conscience 'that modicum of innate science with which each one is born.'

The growth of human conscience, in its perception of justice and in its sympathetic relation to creation, is the surest measure of individual and national progress. Various intellectual theories may be formed as to the origin and growth of conscience. It may be held to be intuitive—springing up as inevitably as the instinctive feelings born with the natural relations of life; or it may be looked upon as gradually evolved—the 'result of countless experiences of fear, love, utility, transmitted through generations.'

But however originating, conscience is a positive and potent fact. It is, indeed, the mightiest factor in social life. It is the great controller of selfhood. It enlarges human character and guides human conduct. The deepening of this principle through the growth of justice and sym-pathy marks an advancement in the type of humanity. Increasing respect for life is one of the clearest signs of growing conscience. Our reverence for the principle of life grows with our enlarging intellectual perception of its universality and its unlimited power of development.

As life is marked by activity, and cannot remain stationary, so conscience shares this law of life. It must inevitably advance or retrograde.

The degradation as well as the development of conscience may be seen amongst us in the midst of our present civilization. It is contrary to the most rudimentary element of conscience to feed upon one's kind, and cannibal tribes who devour their captives represent the lowest type of humanity; even the dogs of the Arctic voyager will endure the slow agony of starvation for days before their human taskmasters can compel them to eat the flesh of their companions. The well-known naturalist, **Mr. W. H. Hudson**, states that wolves, when pressed with hunger, will sometimes devour a fellow-wolf; as a rule, however, rapacious animals will starve to death rather than prey upon one of their own kind.

Yet shipwrecked sailors, even of our own English race, have been known to drink the blood and eat the flesh of their comrades when confronted by starvation.

We find that intelligence may exist without conscience, but the human type changes to a destructive force when this separation takes place. A lamentable example of the social danger created by the destruction or absence of rudimentary conscience amongst us is shown by the betrayal and murder of the little boy Eccles, in Liverpool, for the sake of his clothes, by his two companions of eight and nine years old. There was the deliberate plot to entice him to a pond; the throwing him three times into the water as he scrambled out; the final holding him under water until all struggle had ceased. These facts make a striking, but not unique, object-lesson, showing how intelligence may exist without conscience amongst all our appliances of civilization, and the danger of such separation.

Examples of the social devastation produced by official corruption and business dishonesty are too numerous to be detailed; they are seen in what are called civilized countries—in London, Paris, Rome, and across the ocean. The lack of conscience in public and private transactions creates social misery proportioned to its extent.

Recognising, therefore, that this distinctive principle of conscience is a fact of gradual development, that it grows by the union of the moral with the intellectual elements in our nature, and that the far-reaching consequences for good or evil of vivid or dulled conscience in the individual and the nation are far beyond our power of foresight, a grave responsibility rests upon us in this matter. We are bound to realize that any custom, or method of education, or proposed course of action, that seems to violate the natural instincts of humanity, or is contrary to the present enlightened conscience of any section of our Anglo-American race, demands imperatively the most careful consideration on our part.

II.
CONSCIENCE IN MEDICINE.

EVERY intelligent member of the medical profession will certainly recognise the special value of human conscience in the profession.

The problems which are involved in the practice of the beneficent art, the absolute reliance which the anxious patient is compelled to place in his physician, the helplessness of the poor, who form so large a majority of those who need medical aid, and who are without the defences of wealth and station, show the need of keen moral sense, as well as intelligence, in those who practise the art of medicine.

The very discoveries of medical science enforce this necessity; for the possibility of abuse in the employment of such beneficent agents as anæsthetics and hypnotism, by incompetent or conscienceless operators, is a very serious fact.

The suicides that have taken place after so-called 'successful' operations (as, for example, the production of artificial anus), the pathetic exclamation of poor Montagu Williams, that his brilliant operation had ruined his constitution, and the reckless castrations proved by Dr. Chanu in France, are facts, to be seriously weighed by medical conscience, showing the necessity of restraining too eager experiment.

This special responsibility of the medical profession to society is greatly increased by the fact that the training of a very large section of our intelligent youth during the important years of early manhood rests upon them. The moral as well as intellectual influence exerted by those who guide the college, the hospital, the dispensary, and post-graduate classes, will mould the future action of one of the most influential portions of the community, those, viz., on whom the health of the nation chiefly rests.

Now, whilst all recognise the need of the trained and skilful care of a nation's health, and perceive also that rightly organized medical schools and hospitals are of great value in educating our health guardians, how is it that a profound distrust of these institutions has grown up in our midst; that the support of hospitals becomes increasingly difficult, whilst at the same time the sentiment of benevolence and desire to help the poor is constantly extended?

How is it that the beneficent and necessary art of medicine no longer commands that respect and confidence which its essential character as part of our social institutions would seem to demand?

The answer to these serious questions involves both moral and intellectual considerations. These problems have arisen from failure to perceive that in education moral and intellectual activity cannot be advantageously divorced, or that one portion of our complex nature can be beneficially developed whilst other portions are entirely ignored or injured.

Our medical schools, whilst sharpening the intellectual faculties of their students, are not careful that their modes of teaching bring with them no deterioration of that important faculty of their students, the moral sense. As conscience or the moral sense is unequally developed in human beings, but is indispensable to the physician in his relations with patients, any apathy or negligence in this respect by the trainers of youth may become a national danger.

III.
THE MORAL ELEMENT IN RESEARCH.

MORALITY, as a guide in biological science, is based upon the practical distinction between organic and inorganic Nature.

If medical progress simply involved the investigation of inorganic Nature, the general public would be only learners, gladly receiving such information in geology, chemistry, astronomy, or physics, as specialists in those branches of physical science were good enough to impart to the unlearned.

But directly scientific research passes beyond the distinctive realm of matter, moulded and transformed by general energy, but not affected by individual will, it has to deal with a very different principle, viz., life. This vital distinction has been well laid down by one of our eminent medical authorities as follows: 'During the slow growth of medical knowledge it has become more and more plain that physics, chemistry, and biology are distinct sciences, with methods of their own and inductions of their own; each of the latter terms in the series using the results of its predecessors, and adding new results of its own. Although life is a structure built up of physical and chemical facts, yet to the building, to the arrangement, to the ordering of those facts, there goes something that neither physics nor chemistry can explain, any more than algebra can explain the behaviour of a magnet. To strive to interpret the series of events which make up the life of an animal in terms of chemical change (metabolism), or of conservation or expenditure of energy, is an endeavour which will fail.'

As the brute creation, as well as human beings, share in a physical organization which expresses each variety of life, there is not the same sharply-dividing line between the various categories of animal life as there is between organic and inorganic Nature. Biogenesis, or life generated bylife, is the distinctive feature of organic Nature. We are linked to living creatures of higher or lower nature by the power of educating or subduing them, and by all those varying relations involved in the mystery of life.

The distinctive position of man, as an animal placed at the head of the animal world, necessarily creates serious responsibility on the part of the higher towards the lower creature.

This basis of moral responsibility extends in kind, it not in degree, to all life. It necessitates a directing conscience, which shall guide all our intellectual and practical relations with every category of life.

This moral element enters unavoidably into our treatment of animal life from its lowest to its highest form. Our treatment of a monkey or a prince contains an element of moral attitude which does not exist in our relation to inorganic Nature.

It is a difference of kind as well as of degree, which it is blindness to ignore.

The divergence which now exists between some biological investigators and their critics rests upon the failure to recognise that moral error may engender intellectual error.

The special subject which has produced this controversy is the present method of using the lower animals in biological research, which has so enormously extended of late years. The essence of the controversy is the ethical question, viz.: Have we a right to torture?

It must be distinctly understood that there is here no question of our right under certain circumstances to put to death. Neither is there a doubt of the utility of rational experiment and of research. But the right to put to death in the most humane manner known to us, and the right to torture to death, are two widely different questions.

We have no right, for any purpose whatever, to torture a living creature to death, either by the mutilation of the organs, the slow deprivation of the necessary conditions of life, or the still slower process of destroying by the inoculation of disease.

IV.
RIGHT AND WRONG METHOD.

IT must be carefully noted that the wrong involved in inflicting torture upon a living creature is the violation of a rational principle. The employment of torture or of painful experiment in biological research is not a question of the right to gain knowledge. It is a question of how we seek to gain knowledge. It applies directly to method.

Thus, the fact observed by **Paget**, that in a patient who vomited all fat, the pancreas alone was found on post-mortem examination to be diseased, is worth more than a series of experiments on lower animals of different constitution from our own.

In the slow approach towards truth—which is the great object of science—no single method is indispensable. The human mind is so full of activities; Nature presents such an infinite variety of resources, that progress in research can never be hindered by the choice of right instead of wrong method.

This is well stated by **one of our most experienced investigators** when he says:

'Methods run with the manners and customs of the ages. In science there is no one method that can be considered indispensable. Attributes are indispensable; observation, industry, accuracy are indispensable; methods are not. They may be convenient, they may be useful, they may be expedient, but nothing more.'

This admirable statement throws a flood of light upon the confusion and perplexity of the present controversy. It shows the error of both the so-called unscientific and scientific parties. It shows the error (not unnatural) in the former of confounding together experiment, research, laboratory, and scientific investigation, and classing them under one indiscriminate ban of cruelty; it also shows the narrow vision and false reasoning of those who claim that right and wrong have no meaning when applied to the investigation of phenomena supposed to be revealed by the senses. or state that the collecting of so-called facts, named knowledge, is an end in itself, to be unrestrained and justified in itself.

That interesting book, 'The Naturalist in La Plata,' in narrating the author's observation of the natural fearlessness of all wild animals towards man, the careful research into life-habits that can be carried on where this fearlessness is not betrayed, and the susceptibility to kindness which exists amongst all the lower animals to their sovereign, man, furnishes a striking and delightful suggestion as to the *method* which future research should take.[1]

It is the distinctive moral relation existing in the plane of animal life that makes our connection with the organic world a different and more comprehensive relation than that which exists with inorganic Nature. It places research in the biological sciences on a different plane from study of the physical sciences.

Therefore, whilst it would be folly for ordinary people to criticise the methods of experts in physical science, it would be dastardly dereliction of duty not to consider the methods employed in biological science.

The subject of experimentation upon the lower animals having two aspects—an ethical and an intellectual one—the medical profession will be wise to welcome all honest and kindly criticism and suggestion in the most difficult of all studies, viz., the study of life. It must be recognised that the people are absolutely in their right in refusing to submit to dictation in what concerns their relation to animal life, of which they are the responsible head.

> 1. This sound method is well exemplified in the writings of the French naturalist Le Roy.

V.
THE NECESSITY OF MEDICAL RESEARCH.

WHILST fully recognising the right of the laity to criticise scientific method when it deals with sentient animals, fashioned on the same general plan as ourselves, and capable of fear, pain, affection, and gratitude, there is another aspect of the subject which we are bound to consider.

The present condition of medicine is that of an art, not of a science. It is erroneous to speak of the science of medicine. There exists uncertainty in diagnosis, uncertainty in the action of remedies, ignorance of individual idiosyncrasy, and terrible inability to meet such devastating diseases as cancer, consumption, leprosy, etc.

No one outside the profession can fully realize the grave responsibility, even desperate anxiety, felt by the conscientious physician when life or death seems to depend upon his action, and he knows that medical resources are not equal to the occasion. It is a noble desire for the advancement of the beneficent art of medicine which makes the great body of busy doctors eagerly listen to those who are supposed to speak with authority, and hail with hope every announcement or supposed discovery which seems to promise improved practical results.

This is really a sound humane attitude of mind in that vast body of the profession who are unable, from the pressure of practical life, to devote themselves to investigation—a profession which has always had its heroes and martyrs, who have not shrunk from risking their lives in the service and for the advancement of their noble art.

Those also who are in the profession can most fully estimate the real and beneficial results, both in surgery and medicine, derived from careful and persistent research, notwithstanding the severe disappointment often caused by the theoretical error and unjustifiable practice resulting from rivalry in erroneous methods of investigation. The conquest of pain and diminution of nervous shock in necessary surgical operations[1]; the disappearance of blood-poisoning, hospital gangrene, and erysipelas, which were the scourges of our public institutions in a former generation, are immense gains, due to the discovery of anaesthetics, antiseptics, and advancing sanitation. These blessings are the direct outcome of persevering and skilful clinical observation, of careful work in the laboratory, of humane experiment, and of happy accident; they are not derived from cruel experimentation.

The successful control of that terrible disease—puerperal fever—which formerly destroyed such a multitude of women, is a striking conquest of humane method in modern medicine. When I was a student in La Maternité of Paris in 1849, this destructive malady of lying-in women produced a mortality varying from 10 to 15 per cent. But when I visited La Maternité in 1889 the mortality was reduced to a little over 1 per cent. This was due to rigorous cleanliness, sanitation, and the use of antiseptics, directed by the skilful *sage femme en chef* Madame Henri, in spite of the old and unsuitable buildings and the depressing status of many of the patients.

A still more satisfactory result is shown in Dr. Annie McCall's Clapham Maternity, Where not a single death occurred amongst the 760 cases first received into the institution.

This excellent result still continues under the same administration. In the 2,100 lying-in eases received to date in the hospital, there has been no death from puerperal fever. This excellent record has been attained by scrupulous cleanliness, absolute isolation on the occurrence of suspicious symptoms, by excellent nursing,.and constant oversight by the doctors in charge. Even in the out-patient department, where the conditions of living are not under such strict medical control, the deaths from this frightful malady have only amounted to 4 in 7,000 cases under the same enlightened direction.

This great and beneficent reform in the first and world-wide branch of medicine, by means of which the lives of innumerable women in all our large centres of civilization have been saved, is the result of scientific research. It was initiated and successfully carried out by Semmelweis, of Vienna,[2] and is a striking instance of the value of research carried on by the use of the comparative method, with absolutely no resort to experiment. The history of this reform, the methods by which it was accomplished, the opposition it encountered in the profession itself, and its triumphant vindication, are well worth serious study. An account of this valuable investigation, as also of Pettenkofer's research in cholera (referred to later), and other important discoveries by justifiable methods of inquiry, are given to English readers by the admirable translation published by the New Sydenham Society.

Medical research, therefore, is not only justifiable, but obligatory in a profession that is specially charged with the care and advancement of individual and national health; and, as will be seen later, observation, induction, and rational experiment form the essential methods of scientific inquiry.

These two facts, viz., the necessity of advance in medical knowledge, and the methods of investigation necessary for such advance, must be distinctly recognised by sincere reformers, and should shield the profession from that indiscriminate reproach which is often made against it as a whole; for such hostility tends to strengthen that undue *esprit de corps* which often hinders sound medical progress in the profession.

1. The former horrors of the hospital operating-room are graphically described from personal observation in **Sir B. W. Richardson**'s treatise, 'The Mastery of Pain.'
2. See the standard work of Hirsch on 'Geographical and Historical Pathology,' vol. ii., pp. 416-466. The value of this translation is greatly increased by its excellent index.

VI.
RESTRICTION OF EXPERIMENT.

WHEN we investigate the popular or ethical aspect of so-called scientific research, made upon living animals, we are at once met by facts which imperatively demand both serious thought and determined action, if we would not be participators in the degradation of human conscience. We are confronted with the enormous increase in such experiments which has taken place within the last thirty years, as well as in the severity of the sufferings inflicted. This increase is going on in England as well as in foreign countries.[1] It is growing in many cases, not only without any benefit to the human race, but also without reference to any supposed beneficial result, as its attempted justification.

The volume of facts and evidence collected by Mr. Colam (the able Secretary of the Royal Society for the Protection of Animals), and published by that society in 1876, is a permanent record of great value. It enables us to measure the growth of experimentation in England, not only from 1862 to 1876, when the present Cruelty to Animals Bill was enacted, but it also forms a point of comparison for testing the increase of vivisectional methods since 1876 to the present day, when these easy but often fallacious methods of research have become universal in medical investigation and medical instruction.

In 1869 there were very few places where experimentation on animals could be carried on, such investigations being made by men of rare ability, and for a definite object. There were no class demonstrations, and no students encouraged to experiment. But in 1892 there were 180 persons licensed in this country, and over 3,960 experiments performed, numbers which increase with each year, the amount of unlicensed experiment being of course an unknown quantity, depending on individual conscience.

The Effect on Students and Subordinates.

A point for serious consideration is the effect produced upon the unformed minds of students of medicine, by the introduction of experimentation upon living animals into our medical schools and hospitals.

The employment of destructive experimentation on living creatures is now introduced as a part of the ordinary instruction of medical students in the fundamental study—physiology. This is a novelty of the present generation. During the whole course of my medical studies, forty years ago, I never saw a living creature vivisected for the instruction of students. The same is true of the experience of most of the able physicians of an older generation.

Now, however, every medical school has its store of imprisoned living creatures awaiting their fate—from the large frogs imported from Germany, the mice, rabbits, cats, and dogs of home production, to the cargoes of monkeys brought to our foggy climate from tropical Africa. They form an enormous mass of living creatures, kept for the attempted demonstration of vital action in the lecture-room, or for the study of diseased processes in the physiological laboratory.

It is a fallacy (although proclaimed in high places) that the ordinary student of medicine must be prepared for his practical work as a physician for men by watching the opening of chest, abdomen, brain, or cutting into the delicate vital organs of living lower animals. Such demonstration is a thrilling spectacle to inexperienced students. It appeals to that love of excitement which makes them rush to a surgical operation, or to an extraordinary medical case which may have no bearing whatever on their future practice, whilst the commonplace but all-important bedside observation seems dull in comparison. Yet patient work in the anatomical and microscopic rooms, and in the chemical laboratory for general and animal chemistry, and close clinical study, all of which involve no form of suffering, are of primary importance. The genius of a Professor, as an instructor, is shown by his ability to make his pupils realize this.

Destructive experimentation on helpless animals —not for their own benefit—is a demoralizing practice. The student becomes familiar with the use of gags, straps, screws, and all the paraphernalia of ingenious instruments invented for overpowering the resistance of the living creature. or for guarding the operator from injury in case the anaesthetic, when used, should give out too soon. He learns also how easy it is to experiment in secret.

By advanced instruction and post-graduate classes the student is led on to take active part under licensed authority in this fascinating, but morally dangerous, method of study. Moreover, the large body of subordinates, who are necessary to take charge of and prepare the animals, are trained in indifference to suffering, without any excuse of intellectual gain; and the same injurious influence extends in ever-widening circles—to the traders who invent and sell instruments of torture, and to those who supply the living material.

Now, the natural instinct to be cherished in human beings is protection and kindliness to infancy and all helpless creatures, not indifference to suffering or wilful infliction of it. As human conscience is a thing of growth or degradation, the natural shrinking from needless pain can soon be hardened into callousness. Conversing with medical students, in relation to the effect made upon them by witnessing vivisections, even under chloroform, I have found that their experience is always the same, viz.: first, the shock of repulsion, then tolerance, and then, if often repeated, indifference.

The moral deterioration necessarily induced in those to whom suffering becomes a frequent spectacle is noted by the 'Englishman in Paris,' from personal experience. After speaking of the inhumanity produced by the daily sight of blood, in the originally honest bourgeois, who became the 'Conventionnels' of the French Revolution in 1793, he writes as follows: 'I have witnessed three executions. After Pommeraye's execution, I was ill for a week; after Troppmann's, the effect soon wore off in three days; after Campa's, I ceased to think about it in twenty-four hours. Then I made a vow that no power on earth should draw me to the Place de la Roquette again. But men generally regard their growing imperviousness as a sign of mental force, and pride themselves upon it.'

In Marie Bashkertseff's 'Journal' is a striking passage which describes the effect of a Spanish bull-fight. She says: 'I was able to maintain a tranquil air in full view of the butchery, carried on with the utmost refinement of cruelty. One leaves the scene slightly intoxicated with blood, and feeling desirous to thrust a lance into the neck of every person one meets. I stuck my knife into the melon I was cutting at table, as if it were a banderilla I were planting in the hide of a bull, and the pulp seemed like the palpitating flesh of the wounded animal. The sight is one that makes the knees tremble and the head throb. It is a lesson in murder.'

The moral distinction between heroism shown when suffering is witnessed, for the purpose of aiding the sufferer, and that evinced for the selfish desire of individual gain or excitement, was strikingly exhibited by a German nurse, whom we sent on to the army during the Civil War in America. This frail-looking woman drifted on to the front, and after the Battle of Gettysburg, donning a pair of man's boots, wading in pools of blood and mud, spent two days and nights on the field of slaughter, drawing out still-breathing bodies from the heaps of slain, binding up wounds, giving a draught of water, placing a rough pillow under the head, in an unselfish enthusiasm that knew neither hunger nor fatigue. The ghastly wounds, the blood, the shrieks and groans of that horrid scene, served but as fuel to the fire of humanity that consumed her.

The Effect on Teachers or Practitioners of Medicine.

In considering the subject of experimentation, reason requires that we realize the necessary distinction between the methods employed in training students for a practical profession, and the exceptional position of the few geniuses who possess the rare combination of qualities essential to scientific investigation. In calling attention to this distinction, we do not condone torture; for this can be proved to be unscientific. But it emphasizes a growing and mischievous evil of the present day, when numbers of ordinary teachers of physiology, whose gifts are limited, and whose especial business is to instruct students in the knowledge which has been attained, consider themselves capable of original scientific research, or attempt to repeat before either students or popular audiences so-called demonstrations on living creatures.

The showy plan of experimenting on animals is undoubtedly a great temptation to teachers of somewhat shallow intellect. Such practice readily gains the gratifying applause of inexperienced learners, who are misled by an appearance of conclusiveness in the lectures, which they are quite incompetent to gauge. But the influence thus exercised is a harmful one, diverting the mind from right methods of study.

The temptation to make a display before imperfectly informed persons is too great. If the profession is to advance in popular esteem, it will recognise that the unfeeling destruction of living creatures, even the pithing of a frog or the dissection of the salivary glands of a living mouse, is a false method of forming the minds of students which should be entirely abandoned.

We must here note the demand lately made by some leading members of the profession for increased facilities for experimentation on animals. Now, anyone who studies the Cruelty to Animals Bill (30 and 40 Vict.), which in 1876 licensed vivisection in Great Britain,[2] will see how easy it now is to obtain a license, and how carefully the provisions of the Bill are arranged to give freedom to experimentation—in fact, to protect experimenters rather than their helpless victims. Thus, whilst in Section 2 a penalty of £100 or three months' imprisonment is imposed for acts of cruelty, the Bill proceeds in Section 3 to give absolute freedom to every licensed person to torture, to mutilate, to disease, to any extent if he considers it advisable to do so. In Section II it gives exceeding wide scope for procuring licenses. By Sections 7-10 it makes the efficient oversight of licensed persons almost impossible, and by the provisions of Sections 13-15 it virtually excludes the influence of growing humanity conscience in the community from being exerted on the persons and places licensed. In short, the Bill would rather seem to be skilfully devised to give a free hand to persons who may call themselves 'scientific,' than to protect living creatures who cannot protect themselves.

The plea put forward by the gentlemen referred to, viz., that medical progress is now hindered in England by restrictions, is practically a justification by them of the inhuman practices which prevail in France, Germany, Russia, and the United States, and in all countries where the con-science of the people has not been aroused to the moral and intellectual dangers involved in the torture of animals.[3]

Surely these English physicians who demand entire freedom for vivisection do not realize what the result of foreign methods is. They cannot have noted the innumerable examples of atrocious cruelty which are occurring in the records of medical research, as practised on the Continent and in America.

They cannot have taken note of such typical examples as the utterly useless barbarity of Senn of Philadelphia, setting fire to a dog that he had pumped full of hydrogen gas, before the Medical

Congress of Berlin in 1890. Nor the experiments in massage on a series of large disjointed dogs, performed in Professor Charles Richet's Paris laboratory, not only with the permission, but with the consultative advice, of that gentleman. A set of more unjustifiable experiments were never devised.

Yet these are only examples of frequently occurring atrocities, where vivisection is unchecked. Certainly no body of honourable English physicians who are in the habit of reading *Les Archives Générales de Médecine* would fail to condemn such fallacious experiments, where the pretence of anæsthesia served to diminish the resistance of the victims—not to annihilate pain. Yet such cruelties inevitably result from free vivisection.

Factors in Human Nature.

It must never be forgotten that gambling excitement, or the spirit of undue emulation, exists in all classes of men—in biological investigators as well as others—and it needs guidance, or restraint.

The German officer Reizenstein felt keen remorse for the murder of his beautiful Irish mare Lippespringe, yet he and his companions tortured thirty horses to death under the temporary insanity of intense rivalry. But it was possible to bring public conscience to bear on this barbarity, and thus check the recurrence of any similar future aberration.

So in biological research we see the disastrous effects of individual and national rivalry. They are shown in the contradictory results of false methods of observation, in the endless repetition of similar painful experiments, in the strife of conflicting theories, and in the practical failure of results obtained from the lower animals when applied to the human race.

The moral sense of a noble profession may well be appealed to, to create a conscience which shall check the present grave abuses of so-called research.

> 1. Thus, the authorities of Paris ordered twenty friendless dogs to be tied to the branches of trees in a wood, and a shell made in the municipal laboratory exploded amongst them, riddling and mangling them fearfully.
> 2. The humane and carefully-guarded Bill drawn up by the Royal Society for the Protection of Animals, and introduced by the Earl of Harrowby and Lord Carnarvon, was rejected.
> 3. The judicious remarks of Lord Farrer in relation to municipal affairs apply equally to the subject under consideration. He says: 'My immediate object, however, is not to preach upon the general question, but to make a practical suggestion. What we want to know is, Which of the two ways of doing any particular work is the cheaper and the better? Much experience of public departments leads me to doubt their own reports upon their own doings; not, of course, from any dishonesty on the part of the officials, but from a natural tendency in every man to make the best of what he does. It is for this reason, as well as

from want of sufficient experience, that I cannot feel absolute confidence in the reports made to the London County Council on the results of their own experiments.'

VII.
PRURIGO SECANDI.

ANOTHER serious ethical danger connected with unrestrained experiment on the lower animals is the enormous increase of audacious human surgery, which tends to overpower the slower but more natural methods of medical art, and to divert attention from hygiene.

This modern increase of surgery, entailing permanent mutilation, has received a special name, prurigo secandi, or cacoethes secandi. It prevails in France, and in every country where no restraint is placed on animal experimentation,[1] or where the importance of not injuring the moral sense of students has not been recognised.

The great increase in ovariotomy, and its extension to the insane, is so notable a result of this prurigo secandi that it becomes a serious question whether the practice of ovariotomy, though sometimes beneficent, is not on the whole a disastrous discovery, and whether it should not be regarded as a confession of medical impotence, of insanitary education and social corruption, rather than as a satisfactory triumph of surgical skill. The destruction of motherhood is either a martyrdom or a degradation. In no case can it be boasted of as 'brilliant surgery.'

Dr. Chanu, in his carefully prepared thesis of 1896, in exposing the grave abuse of this branch of surgery, estimates that there were 500,000 castrated women in France, and one in every 250 women throughout Europe. He finds the decrease of the birth-rate to coincide with the abuse of ovariotomy. 'Dr. Chanu affirmed, before a jury unable to refute his assertion, that the abuse of ovariotomy has done more harm to France in ten years than the Prussian bullets did in 1870, and that the causes of the depopulation of France are closely allied to the practice of the castration of women.'

The prevention of disease in the organs of generation must be sought for persistently in improved education of the young—the male as well as the female—and in JUST relations of the sexes.'

Operative surgery should excite strong suspicion when it enables a Dr. Keppler to exalt 'marriage with a castrated woman as the ideal of a neo-Malthusian union, the only way of securing its object without endangering health and happiness.'[2]

Of the same nature as the prurigo secandi of medical practice is the motive or source of much of the laboratory experimentation.

The various ethical dangers resulting from conscienceless or irrational experiments on animals demand much more serious consideration by the profession than has hitherto been given to them. In the opinion of an increasing number of intelligent physicians, a vast amount of what is now presumptuously called research—experiments disguised under learned names, but which are really the irrational mutilating and diseasing of sentient living creatures—are no more scientific research than is the gratification of a child's curiosity when it sticks a pin, with a thread, through a cockchafer, to see how long it will fly and how loud it will buzz. The child, when punished for its thoughtless cruelty, might remonstrate in learned terms that it should not be restrained, for it was investigating the vital endurance of the *Melolontha vulgaris*, and the acoustic properties of its wing-covers, under interesting and abnormal conditions.

A large proportion of what is simply conscienceless curiosity, often starting from more or less frivolous tentative diversions of the laboratory, though now by courtesy named research, is no more valuable than the child's spinning of the cockchafer, and should be as sharply checked.

The genesis of discovery in biology, with its necessary relations to therapeutics, has yet to be written. Extending experience is more and more clearly showing us, as a practical fact, that whilst observation and rational—*i.e.*, humanely limited—experiment are legitimate and noble efforts for the attainment of improved medicine, cruel and merely curious experiment, condemned by our moral faculties, are misleading and mischievous.

Men like Professor Henschel, of Upsala, and Professor Pettenkofer, of Munich, warn our eager young investigators against drawing conclusions as to human beings from experiments made on animals.

We find, as a matter of fact, that all the *permanent* advances of medicine have been gained whilst pursuing rational and righteous methods; whilst all the fiascoes of supposed discovery have resulted through departing from them.

Anæsthetics, antiseptics, and sanitation are not the result of cruel experimentation.

Danger of Inoculation.

The most serious fallacy arising from erroneous methods of biological research is the practice of vitiating human blood, by the introduction of the diseased products of animals. This dangerous method, which threatens to undermine national health, is the necessary outcome of diseasing animals, on the plea of seeking remedies for human disease.

The intellectual fallacy involved in this practice will be considered later; but its ethical character as affecting conscience must here be noted, as it is this line of research which is productive of the most extended form 0t cruelty to the lower animals, viz., slow torture.

The following extract from records of the Belgian Academy of Medicine illustrates this subject: 'Researches on the inoculability of cancer ought to be encouraged. The numerous experiments made on animals are still contradictory in results. Drs. Francotte and De Rector have, in the years 1891–92, inoculated mice under the skin of the shoulder.

The inoculations were carried on from June, 1891, to May, 1892, when the following appearances were presented: The whole region of the shoulder was inflamed; there was necrosis of the corresponding upper extremity, which dropped off from dry gangrene; the stump left was indurated, hard, and painful, whilst the lymphatic glands in connection with the part were enlarged. The examination of the tumour disclosed nothing very particular. The bones were the seat of osteoperosis, and the arteries showed arteritis. The investigators believe the tumours were cancerous, but this statement must be received with caution.'

Such long-continued torture, even of a mouse, is morally degrading, and, as if in retribution, is doomed to be useless.

A Chinese medical author—Tuan Mei—writing in the last century, 1716–1797, lays down a true medical axiom when he marks the difference between death and torture as follows: 'Living creatures are for our use, and we may put them to death. But we may not make death a boon, and then withhold it from them.'

> 1. 'Professor Leon le Fort, Professor Verneuil, Professor Duplay, and Professor Tillaux, have been asked by a public journal for their opinions on the operative mania (*furie opératoire*), said to be prevalent at present. Professor Le Fort says it is much more widespread in France than in other countries, and in a long letter he protests against the

Custom amongst the young French surgeons, in order to bring their names before the public, "to seek out some operation unknown in France, then seek out a victim on whom they can perform it, in order to report it before a medical society, and perhaps also show the patient." Then, says M. le Fort, they take up the operation as a speciality, perform it on 100 or 200 patients, and thus gain a reputation. Professor Verneuil protests against the abuse of operations in general, and especially of gynaecological operations. He deplores the prurigo secandi with which so many of the French surgeons are attacked. Professor Duplay and Professor Tillaux express the same opinions.' See *Medical Reprints*, May, 1893.

2. See the *Journal de Médecine de Paris.*

VIII.
WHAT IS SCIENTIFIC RESEARCH?

THE apparent opposition between popular and medical judgment in relation to certain methods of biological research, which claim to be scientific, necessitates a clearer knowledge of what science is, and a recognition of the methods of research which can alone be called scientific.

It is certain that knowledge of truth must reconcile varying but honest opinions, and furnish plans of investigation that neither shock the humane development of our nature nor hinder our intellectual progress towards truth.

The terms 'science' and 'scientific' are constantly used and abused. They are often applied to the accumulating of facts or of phenomena; but such accumulation is not necessarily science, and may even hinder science. For although the collecting of facts may bring together valuable materials essential for future use, it may also bring together rotten or sham materials, which will interfere with sound work. A faulty method of endeavouring to obtain facts may seriously destroy the value of the phenomena thus observed.

The gratification simply of intellectual activity or curiosity must not be confounded with genuine research. Curiosity is the outcome of ignorance.

Now, our ignorance of much in Nature is no reproach to anyone; but the way in which curiosity is gratified marks the difference between the simple child and the rational adult. In the childish development curiosity, though useful, is superficial and short-sighted; it is necessarily a shallow impulse which cannot realize the wide relations of existence, and its satisfaction has no necessary connection with the acquisition of valuable knowledge. But the adult rises into a higher plane of thought. Curiosity is no longer unduly exercised, but has grown into a love of truth. It has become that reverential use of reason which is the basis of truth, and which forms the true guide to the attainment of scientific knowledge; for rational method does not isolate a fact from all its connections, but sees it in its relations, and in due proportion. Thus only can valuable knowledge be acquired.

Neither is analysis science. It is only when the observations of analysis are corrected and proved by synthesis that the truth of science can be obtained.

A clear recognition of the different use of analysis and of synthesis is essential in any claim of research to be called scientific. 'Although by analysis we separate, and by synthesis we combine, yet in the synthesis there is more than in all the parts taken analytically. The mere synthesis introduces something entirely new.'

Kant, in speaking of the use of analysis and synthesis in logic, lays down the test of all scientific inquiry. He says: 'Analysis is the first and chief requirement in making our knowledge distinct. For the more distinct our knowledge of a thing is, the stronger and more effective it can be; only the analysis must not go so far that at last the object itself disappears.'

Truth being a unity, the science which demonstrates it must correlate all knowledge.

Science is not, therefore, an accumulation of isolated facts, or of facts torn from their natural relations. To know a thing scientifically is to know it in just relation to all other things. For science unites, and demands the exercise of our various faculties, as well as of our senses.

Science is proved knowledge. It is the study of causes and their relations applied to facts; but such proof can only be obtained by search which is in accordance with the laws of Nature—laws which are gradually discovered by our race.

Natural law is deduced from all the facts of human experience. In searching for and collecting which we must recognise the conditions under which we are placed, the limitations of the present phase of our intellectual powers, the gradual growth of conscience.

Science being proved truth, scientific method requires that all the factors which concern the subject of research shall be duly considered, in order to arrive at correct thought respecting the special subject of inquiry.

The application of scientific method necessarily varies, therefore, according to the subject under investigation.

Thus, the construction of a bridge and the calculation of an eclipse equally involve the bases of scientific method, viz.: observation, deduction, and experiment; but each subject requires a special application of scientific method, suited to the varying nature of the subject of study.

Consequently, biological research, in order to be scientific, requires a special modification of method, because the new factors of sensation and consciousness come into play in biology—factors which do not exist in astronomy, or geology, in mechanics, physics, or chemistry.

In order to attain truth respecting biology, therefore, the facts concerning sensation and consciousness, and their relation with, or the way in which these new factors modify the facts of, physics and chemistry, must be carefully considered in this higher state, which we call life, or the investigation is not scientific, no matter how interesting as an intellectual exercise.

When first endeavouring to find a recognised definition of the term 'science,' I consulted the latest 'Encyclopædia Britannica' of our public library, thinking that from such an acknowledged authority a correct statement could there be obtained. To my surprise, I found that the word 'science' was not included in the list of subjects. Searching further in this record of nineteenth-century thought, under the head of 'Biology'—that department which is ordinarily supposed to be the science of life, as distinguished from the consideration of non-living things—the following principle was found to be laid down, viz., that there was no essential difference between organized and unorganized Nature, for life was simply a property of matter.

It is well to weigh the argument for this doctrine, which necessarily destroys the essential idea of right and wrong, and removes the foundation of good and evil. It is set forth in the following manner:

'The abstract-concrete sciences are mechanics, physics, chemistry.... Whilst their subject-matter is found in a consideration of varied concrete phenomena, they do not aim at a determination of certain "abstract" quantitative relations and sequences known as "laws," which never are manifested in a pure form, but always are inferred, by observation and experiment upon complex phenomena, in which the abstract laws are disguised by their simultaneous interaction.... These sciences of mechanics, physics, and chemistry have for their object to explain concrete phenomena, by reference to the properties of matter set forth in their generalizations.'

The following important dictum in regard to biology is thus laid down:

'It is the business of those occupied with that branch to assign living things in all their variety to the one set of forces recognised by the physicist and chemist... and its evolution' (that is, the evolution of life) 'as the necessary outcome of those forces—the automatic product of those same forces.... The discovery of the mechanical principle of evolution completed the doctrine' (of the material origin of life). '... It may be said to comprise the history of man, sociology, and psychology, viz., the survival of the fittest in the struggle for existence.'

This ignoring by the 'Encyclopædia Britannica' of any definition of the word 'science,' and also the attempted reduction of life to a property of matter, is, however, too limited a view of Nature to be accepted by many thoughtful students of the present day. Turning, therefore, to 'Chambers's Cyclopaedia,' which is the latest expression of the views of the able thinkers of North Britain, an explanation of the term 'science' was found, which is far truer to advancing thought. The comprehensive definition is there given that science 'is the correlation of all knowledge.'

As science searches for causes with their relations, and is proved knowledge, so no branch of knowledge or method of acquiring knowledge can be considered scientific which contradicts any facts of Nature, or which bases its methods on the destruction of those facts.

Truth can only he arrived at by considering various or apparently opposite aspects of human problems; so biological facts, or the problems of organized or living creatures, must be considered, not simply from the side of 'mechanics, physics, and chemistry, or the automatic action of the forces of matter,' but also from the equally positive facts of life, and the forces which careful observation is gradually showing to be enfolded in the fact of mind as developed through protoplasm onward. The facts of affection, companionship, sympathy, justice, are positive forces. They exercise a powerful influence over the physical organization of all living creatures.

These mental forces can change the action of the bodily functions in the most surprising manner, arresting the heart's action, interfering with secretion, or changing natural secretion into poison, and destroying the normal and beneficial controlling action of the nervous system. They are proved by experience to be so striking that they cannot be overlooked in any unprejudiced investigation of natural forces.

A fit of passion in a nursing mother has destroyed her infant; the industrious cultivator, seeing his field of strawberries, the products of his toil, carried off by thieves, has fallen dead in his vain efforts to stop the cruel depredation. But such instances are world-wide, and corroborated by everyone's experience. They prove that, although the force of mechanics, physics, and chemistry are employed in the animal economy, there are also powers far beyond these limited forces, which must be studied also in biological research, if we are to learn how these physical may be overridden by mental forces. Without such correlation of knowledge we fail to realize the unity of Nature, and cannot attain to true science or proved knowledge.

It is thus seen that, as already stated, in useful scientific investigation, the object to be attained, the method to be employed, and the application to be made of the knowledge searched for, must all be considered in determining the distinction between genuine science and simple unguided intellectual activity or curiosity.

It is necessary to emphasize the fact, because this vital distinction is often overlooked in the claim now made for the grand term 'science.'

In defining the meaning and scope of science as pursued by rational beings, it must be recognised as a fundamental principle, which cannot be too often dwelt upon, that what we can do, is not a measure of what we ought to do. Thus, when Stanley attempted to excuse the infamous action of his naturalist, Jameson,[1] by saying that he was a real good fellow, but 'his science misled him,' he degraded the term 'science' by applying it to an act of morbid curiosity.

Again, when the Russian nobleman purchased a child and condemned it to be brought up with a deaf and dumb nurse, under the unnatural condition of deprivation of all social relations, his action was not scientific, but a gratification of inhuman curiosity.

It is within our power apparently to drown an animal, human or brute, and recover it to life again and again, but we gain no scientific knowledge by so doing. We torture the creature and violate our natural instincts, but we acquire no practical benefit to human welfare; on the contrary, we endanger the mental integrity of the experimenter.

It is a short-sighted and hopeless attempt to do violence to Nature in a search for scientific truth. Distinction must be made between the possible and impossible in the conditions under which we are placed in life. Thus, we cannot destroy the family relation, but we can make it happy and conducive to the welfare of the race. We cannot change the method of human generation, but we can Spiritualize its exercise. We cannot destroy the instinct of private property, but we can guide and limit it. We cannot change structure, but we can educate it; nor abolish curiosity, but we can restrain and direct it; nor check invention, but it need not be applied to evil purposes. Neither can we make races equal, but we can establish justice and mercy in the relations of the stronger to the weaker.

This study of the natural laws, which necessarily limit rational human action, applies with especial force to biological research, and explains the reason for limiting scientific method.

Thus, the study of living creatures under unnatural or destructive conditions, although it may be a well-meaning attempt to acquire knowledge, is nevertheless a dangerous one. It is intellectually a false method, which may lead to practical error, and produce a labyrinth of confusion and contradictory experience which hinders the attainment of exact knowledge. It is morally a false method, because it injures those elementary instincts of justice and mercy by whose evolution civilization advances. Thus the progress of the race is retarded.

The present astounding multiplication of drugs, of inoculations, of mutilations in the practice of medicine, with the eager attempt to prove each new invention by a formidable array of imperfect statistics, is a striking object-lesson in the present day, of the error into which false methods of research have led many members of a noble and humane profession. It is a fallacy necessarily proceeding from a wrong view of what science really is.

Although this erroneousness is by no means solely connected with vivisectional methods, yet if the high claim which the noble art of medicine makes to advance our social well-being be justly founded, a stringent obligation rests upon it not to injure the moral sense of its members by the methods employed in education or in practice.

> 1. This naturalist, when amongst cannibals in the Emin Pasha Expedition, bribed the cannibal tribe to eat a young negro girl.

IX.
THE AXIOM OF SCIENCE.

THE fundamental law, without whose observance reliable biological investigation is impossible, is stated as follows:

'In studying the laws alike of organic and of inorganic Nature, the experimenter must be careful not to destroy the phenomenon that is being investigated.'

Intellectual error, as well as practical danger, arises from the attempt to transfer to man results supposed to be gained by fallacious experimentation on the lower animals. The fallacy consists in noting general resemblance of structure, but not the far more remarkable differences of function. If, for instance, the life-habits of two dogs of good breed are closely studied, it will be seen that, although certain individual differences are observed between the dogs, yet they are as nothing when compared with the enormous variation of function between the dog and the human being. The bones and garbage swallowed without injury, and the licking of its body, show the different type of digestion and assimilation, the action of the kidneys, of the various senses, and the possession of senses which we are unable to appreciate; in short, its distinctive type of existence proves the impossibility of drawing safe inferences for man from the digestive or other canine functions. Again, observation and rational experiment, solely for the benefit of one species of animal, may incidentally lead to the benefit of other races of animals; but direct experiment on one type, for the supposed benefit of another kind, is unscientific.

It is this error that vitiates the famous postulates of **Professor Koch**, through the system of 'controls,' the latest exemplification of this fallacy being the attempt to prove the existence of cholera in man by cultivating the bacilli in animals. The same error also produces the failure of **M. Pasteur** to prevent hydrophobia in man.

It is well known how the influence of what we term 'mind' governs the action of the bodily functions, either promoting or disturbing their normal condition. This is a fact of growing importance in practical medicine. Similar influence is exerted in varying degrees on all living creatures. Destructive or non-natural experimentation on living animals is always subject to the fallacy of morbid condition.

The established law of research stated above exposes the error of pursuing biological investigation (or the study of vital action) by the process of mutilating or diseasing living animals.

In research the radical difference between inorganic and organic Nature cannot be too clearly insisted on. Whilst in the former we can resolve compounds into their elements, and recombine them, such process is impossible in organic

Nature. We can take a steam-engine or a watch to pieces, examine their parts, repair them, and put them together again, thus proving our knowledge in this realm of Nature. But a living thing cannot be treated in the same way. Not only the difference of animal type forbids destructive method of investigation, but as the type rises in the scale of creation the growing fact of individual idiosyncrasy increases the uncertainty of erroneous method.

Therefore, the law of scientific research. which forbids the destruction of phenomena to be studied, is profoundly true.

If this law be not observed, intellectual activity may be gratified, self-conceit or love of novelty and excitement may be pandered to, the panic of fear in human beings may be worked upon, but the attainment of scientific truth in biology will be impossible.

It is thus seen that methods of biological research which involve cruel or destructive experimentation are both ethically unjustifiable and intellectually fallacious. They are unscientific methods, which will inevitably be abandoned as we attain to clearer views of that unity of truth in which the reconciliation of human conscience with intellectual activity becomes alone recognised as science.

X.
RATIONAL EXPERIMENT IN RESEARCH.

As an illustration of legitimate and even heroic experiment, the trial made with cholera bacilli by Dr. Von Pettenkofer, of Munich, on himself, during the cholera epidemic of 1891, deserves permanent record.[1] It is of importance as showing the fallacy that may be involved in the exaggerated search for bacilli, as the chief cause of disease, which is the favourite theory and practice of the present day.

Dr. Von Pettenkofer (in opposition to the common medical belief) asserts that the diffusion of the cholera germ or cholera bacillus is not the chief cause of cholera. He states that there are two other absolutely necessary conditions, without which no outbreak of cholera is possible; and if these conditions are not present, the cholera germ may be breathed with no production of cholera.

The first condition is the unhealthy state of the soil or locality. But even this does not produce an outbreak if the second condition does not exist, viz., individual predisposition; and he shows that neither the cholera germ nor the insanitary locality, nor both combined, will produce cholera if this individual predisposition does not exist. He further states that no experiments upon the lower animals can be relied on; the only *proof* in relation to cholera must be from the experience of human beings.

The supremacy of sanitation is the lesson which is being gradually taught by such humane scientific experiments. Dirt in its largest sense asmatter in the wrong place, whether in air, water, food, clothing, habitation, soil, or contact, is undoubtedly a main physical cause of disease.

But in all epidemic disease the emotion of fear must be recognised as a most potent predisposing cause. The great fact of mind or emotion is a powerful influence in producing, in preventing, or in curing disease.

This psychological side of medicine is only beginning to receive due attention. As the fallacies which arise in animal experimentation from the production of fear, pain, and coma have not yet been fully recognised, so the inevitable influence of mind in modifying physical conditions has never yet been studied scientifically in human medicine. Yet facts exist in unsuspected abundance which need to be collected, verified, tabulated, and their laws of action diligently studied.

It is known that even that strong muscle the heart may be ruptured by the agony of intense emotion. At Blackburn, the daughter of a woman charged with theft became dumb with horror at her mother's sudden arrest. Dr. Gayet, after vainly treating a very pronounced aneurism of the internal carotid artery, was proceeding to operate, when his patient suddenly recovered. Hydrophobia, cholera, and even small-pox, appear to have been caused by fear.

The extent to which even the so-called microbes of infectious diseases may be produced by fear acting on idiosyncrasy demands very serious investigation; for as it is now generally conceded that morbid micro-organisms do not exist *ab ætero*, it is essential to know by what unhealthy conditions the micro-organisms, or living particles that always surround us, become disease germs.

One of our most distinguished London physicians has full records of the following noteworthy case, which is given not as scientifically proved, but as indicating a line of research which it is folly to ignore or refuse to investigate.

This gentleman attended a patient some years ago in an attack of confluent small-pox under these remarkable circumstances: This patient had always exhibited a morbid horror of the disease, refusing to hear anything about it, or to allow it to be referred to in his presence. A friend on one occasion brought a very fine collection of anatomical plates to show him, sent over from France. Amongst them was a representation of confluent small-pox in a woman. No sooner had this gentleman beheld it than he cried, 'Take it away. I cannot look at it; it makes me ill!' The next day his son sent for the doctor to see his father, who had felt unwell ever since the shock of seeing the pathological plate. He was found suffering from the first symptoms of an illness which proved to be an attack of confluent small-pox. The most searching inquiry failed to discover any traces of the disease, either in the neighbourhood or in any connection whatever with the patient. The cause of this illness, one of the most severe cases the doctor had ever met with, remained a mystery.

It has become of vital importance to investigate 'how far the mental attitude determines or permits the onset of infectious disease.'

> 1. The entirely negative results of all experiments made upon the lower animals to determine if cholera is communicable, or where the poison resides, is demonstrated by an endless series of experiments on the lower animals made in many countries. The extent and severity of these experiments, as well as their inconclusiveness, is impartially detailed in the classic work of Hirst, translated by Dr. C. Creighton, vol. i., in the treatise on 'Asiatic Cholera.'

XI.
THE RANGE OF PAINLESS RESEARCH.

'I AM content to let Nature do all the torturing, and man all the relieving.... The grandest physiology and physiological discovery exist outside every shade of painful experiment.'[1]

These are the words of one of our wisest physicians, deliberately written in the full maturity of a life devoted to original research and its practical application to medicine. His experience led him to the recognition of this great truth: that the supreme aim of the medical profession must become more and more the advancement of sanitation. In any comprehensive view of medical art as a science, the cure of disease is rationally secondary to its prevention.

This, notwithstanding the trade exigencies of competitive living, is recognised by the established rule of the profession, that the physician's first duty is not to injure his patient.

Sanitation necessarily takes into consideration all the elements, both mental and physical, of our complex nature.

It is by the investigation of the laws of healthy created life and their practical application that progress in medicine must be looked for. By observing 'scientifically' the method and variations of these laws, we shall approach nearer to the understanding of 'vital force.'

An immense range of biological inquiry urgently invites the genius of those who are gifted with the rare power of original research.

This range is practically unlimited. The collection of all useful or suggestive facts gathered by genuinely scientific methods from the enormous accumulations to be found in our Government reports, in the records of our medical periodic literature, in the observations of hospitals, societies, cliniques, and private practice, would, if properly arranged and tabulated, form a most useful branch of such a centre. If such collection and examination were extended to the records of other countries, the value as well as labour of the work would be greatly increased.

The observation of the dietetic and hygienic as well as medical treatment of disease, including climate, soil, atmospheric conditions, the distribution of disease, the effect of occupations, pre-natal influences, and later training, are essential.

The action of mineral waters, of compressed and medicated air, the hydration of tissues, the conversion of vegetable into animal tissue, the action of the various constituents of the human body as curative of disease, present necessary subjects of investigation.

A careful judicial inquiry into the claims of specific cures, where a sufficient case for investigation is presented (as *Echinacea augustifolia* in snake-bite, also the Russian bath as preventive of hydrophobia), would form another valuable department.

In fact, it is impossible to specify the full range of important subjects which demand the devotion of able and painstaking research, working upon the careful study of each type of life for the benefit and improvement of that type.

In no branch of this wide range of inquiry is painful experiment necessary.

Our homes, our industrial occupations, our legislative enactments, should all be guided by hygienic knowledge, and its diffusion should be actively encouraged by the community. Our hospitals and dispensaries need to promote practical hygiene. Our medical schools should turn the force of their learning ability and great influence to the conversion of their students into a vast body of sanitary missionaries. If our thousands of medical graduates turned out every year into practice could go forth inspired with enthusiasm for health, convinced that the preservation of health was their especial work, and that all disease must be regarded as a violation of the laws of health, a violation which it was their special duty to fight against; a mighty step in the advancement of medicine would be taken. The impulse to such progress should come from improved instruction in our medical schools, and in the management of our hospitals.

We much need also an unprejudiced and exhaustive history of the progress of biological inquiry since the Middle Ages, with its present result in therapeutics. Such a history may be expected to confirm the not unfounded opinion that the most important advances in practical medicine have been made by methods which are not in any way at variance with our natural instincts of justice and mercy.

> 1. See 'Biological Experimentation,' by **Sir B. W. Richardson**. Bell and Sons.

XII.
RECAPITULATION OF PRINCIPLES.

I. THE attainment of truth, not the gratification of curiosity or of personal ends, is the sole and distinctive aim of genuine scientific research.

II. It is a radical intellectual error to apply the same methods of investigation, suitable to inorganic facts, to the study of organic facts. Natural law being mind ruling matter, every method employed in research into organic Nature must respect and take into account the inseparable mental factor in each type of sentient life, or it becomes unscientific, and may promote fallacy, not truth. Destructive experiment on living creatures, even under the partial suspension of consciousness produced by anæsthetics, is an erroneous method, producing confused or contradictory results.

III. Scientific research in biology must be based upon close and extensive observation of the varying forms of animal life, under natural conditions, with post-mortem examination of the records left by health and disease. Experiments, whether for the repair of lesions or the cure of disease, can only become scientific when made upon the type of life to be benefited by the experiment.

IV. Any experimentation which creates involuntary suffering in living creatures vitiates the necessary conditions of scientific research, and tends to degrade human conscience by producing indifference to suffering.

V. In training our future practitioners of the healing art, the cultivation of respect for life, and the strengthening of enlightened sympathetic conscience in dealing with all poor or helpless creatures, are of paramount importance. The present system of medical education requires revision in order to make health, not disease, the central subject of study.

Finally, full and generous encouragement to those who are engaged in important painless research is urgently needed. Such research should be carried on, if possible, in connection with the great body of serious scientific investigations, by persons of proved ability and clear moral sense, and the work should be cordially open to the observation of all earnest friends.

Such research, reconciling by right methods of investigation intellectual activity with human conscience, would increase our knowledge and advance our well-being in accordance with the higher reason of the race. Only when thus guided by intelligence and conscience can biological research deserve the noble name of science.

APPENDIX

DR. VON PETTENKOFER proceeded to experiment on himself, choosing Munich, in daily communion with Hamburg (where the epidemic was raging), as the place of operations, and sent to Hamburg for the cholera germs. On October 7 he swallowed a centimetre of fresh cholera culture in the presence of witnesses—*i.e.*, infinitely more than could be taken in by touching the lips with contaminated fingers, a cubic centimetre of culture being calculated as containing a thousand million microbes. He in no way changed his manner of living, eating accustomed food, including fruit, cucumbers, and other forbidden articles of diet. During the following week his physiological condition, pulse, temperature, etc., were carefully noted. Nothing unusual occurred but a little internal rumbling and slight diarrhoea, which passed away of itself. Two skilled bacteriologists, MM. Peiffer and Emerich, carefully examined the secretions during this experiment.

M. Von Pettenkofer himself thus states the results:

'The comma bacilli not only prospered in my digestive tube, but had so multiplied in it, that it was evident they found a congenial soil. They were found there in quantities, and in a state of pure culture. But on October 14 all the secretions were normal, only containing a few isolated microbes, which had entirely disappeared on the 18th.

'Now, most bacteriologists assert that the cholera bacilli 'remaining in the intestines secrete there a poison, which, being absorbed, produces the cholera. But what a quantity of poison must have been secreted by these milliards of bacilli during the eight days' sojourn in my intestines! Yet I felt perfectly well, had an excellent appetite, felt neither indigestion nor fever, etc., and I attended every day to my usual occupations. Whence I conclude that the comma bacillus, though it 'may cause a little diarrhoea, produces neither European nor Asiatic cholera.

'Now, it must not be imagined that I am the adversary of the cholera bacillus; but it is erroneous to suppose that when a specific microbe has been discovered in the secretions of an infectious disease that the means of fighting it has also been discovered. The discovery of the bacillus of consumption was just as interesting as the discovery of the cholera bacillus, but since its discovery phthisis has destroyed neither one man less nor one man more.

'These (bacteriological) methods for protection against cholera rest purely upon theory; and it seems to be thought that henceforth cholera, etc., ought to behave according to the prevalent theory, instead of theory being modified according to the cholera. Instead of trying to catch the comma bacillus and draw a cordon around it, the essential thing is to make all the dwelling-places of man healthy.'

Such is the vigorous and genuinely-scientific experiment of a distinguished medical investigator.

Other experimenters have confirmed Dr. Von Pettenkofer's observations. On October 17 Dr. Emerich made a similar experiment on himself, with like results.

Since then, experiments have been made in the Vienna Pathological Institute, with the following results: Six persons partook of the comma bacillus in no mean quantity, and not one of them has had the disease. The six are two doctors, the servant of the Institute, two medical students, and a private gentleman. Professor Stricker treated them all. Two did not feel their health impaired at all; one had headache, was slightly feverish, and could not sleep; two had slight attacks of diarrhoea; and only one was really ill, but recovered at the end of a week. These experiments inspire medical men with serious misgivings as to the theory which considers the comma bacillus as the cause of all cholera.

It is by the recognition of this true method of biological research, and by the generous support of physiologists who honestly seek for truth, even when opposed by temporary fashions of medical opinion, that medicine will become a science.

www.ingramcontent.com/pod-product-compliance
Lightning Source LLC
Chambersburg PA
CBHW061217180526
45170CB00003B/1040